Dedicated
To Your
Awakened Mind

Confronting Cancer
With Greater Awareness

A Survivor's Handbook
(A Basic Understanding)

Table of Contents

I. Introduction

The context of this book applies to all forms of cancer, with a section on head and neck occurrences. You're invited to take this content to heart, from mine to yours, and be clear that what you're about to read is solely the perspective of one human being and his gained knowledge. As in science, we do our best to live in the inquiry and not the findings, as they frequently change.

Head and neck cancer includes areas from the brain to the bottom of the neck, i.e. the mouth, throat, voice box, nasal cavity, sinuses, salivary and lymph glands. Common symptoms are either visual swelling and lumps or internal occurrences that are sometimes initially undetectable. Early detection can make it easier to alleviate metastasis as well as a death sentence.

The risk of getting head and neck cancer increases because of alcohol consumption, tobacco use, breathing in toxic fumes, and chronic infections.[1] To date, the medical treatment typically involves surgery, radiation, and/or chemotherapy. Head and neck cancer is highly curable if treated early, although life expectancy and quality of life depend on certain conditions that will be shared in this handbook.

Cancer therapies, notably radiation therapy,[2] wreak extended havoc on the human body, no matter what cancer type is being treated. In this handbook, there is more focus on head and neck cancer because it remains the most life-challenging after treatment is complete. The reason is that radioactive fibrosis continues to infiltrate living cells and modern medicine has not yet found a way to stop it. The migration of radiation continues to create more fibrotic tissue, creating an array of health challenges.

There's still so much more that we don't know that *we don't know*, and also know that *we don't know*, yet we live our lives thinking that we know; how foolish are we? This often applies to the totality of our lives as well. However, when it pertains to practicing medical science on human beings, it underscores that acts of kindness and a commitment to do little harm remain the focus. Radiation protocols of the future must either continue to be reduced in intensity or completely excluded as a treatment option. Patients who have lived past the radiation life expectancy of head and neck cancer (estimated at 0 - 8 years, having been administered 3000-7000 rads of radiation, depending on the intensity of the protocol), are not usually followed up on by oncologists after eight years and are left to fend for themselves.

II. The Intention of this Handbook

This handbook is intended to empower you, the reader. Being fully responsible for creating our health and well-being is easy to comprehend, however, becoming responsible for having created your dis-ease, is another story because it's not something the average person wants to tackle or even admit.

With so much yet to learn about health and dis-ease, this handbook might help upgrade awareness and allow survivors to thrive in a *new normal* lifestyle change. From the moment you became aware of having the big 'C', until now, your life has not been the same, nor will it for the rest of your days. That said, the good news is that you will soon learn that only you have the option to create a healthier life for yourself.

Many of us still harbor fear and stigma around cancer, so first, it may be best to understand some basic aspects of the human body to diminish the remainder of your fears.

<u>A Basic Understanding of Your Body's Energetic Tendencies</u>[3]

Unless your body is in perfect form, which no one's body usually is, from the time you are born, some areas are energetically weaker than others. To understand and become more aware of this, do your best to recall any patterns of past illnesses you have had that seem to have centered around the same area(s). It may take some focused analysis to realize this area(s)

For example, if you currently have or have had head and neck cancer, look to see how many times you've had issues with the area in which your cancer was located. Chances are, this area has energetically been a weakened spot for some time. These areas are the most vulnerable to disease. Most of us are asleep to our body's energetics because we are not taught to give our bodies this kind of attention. Meditation, quieting down, and being still are ways to become familiar with the energetics of our body and mind. This is the doorway to paying greater attention to the smaller nuances of our energy weaknesses. In addition, the knowledge gained gives us the tools to strengthen those areas.

In a book written by Louise Hays called "You Can Heal Your Life"[4], she attempted to cover all areas in the human body, concerning their weakness, the beliefs that may have caused the dis-ease, along with suggesting new perspectives to put in place to help them heal. Keep in mind that any mental or emotional dis-ease, can energetically manifest into disease.

Understanding the body from an energetics point of view isn't airy-fairy whatsoever. Martial artists, yogis, mentalists, and many folks devoted to holistic health are quite efficient at this. Sadly, they happen to be in the minority.

Take, for example, Bruce Lee, the famous martial artist. He could tell simply by sensing the heat and sound energy of his opponent's body when the person was close enough for him to kick back his foot and hit them square in the jaw without needing to look. This requires mastery of energetic sensitivity, which came after he had learned the physical requirements needed to obtain a black belt.

Teaching yourself to be more sensitive to the energetics of your body isn't difficult, although it takes a little time. For instance, if you spend only 5 minutes a day energetically exploring your less dominant arm, you'll become more aware of your abilities to scan your entire body. Roll up your sleeves and keep your watch or jewelry on to do this. Close your eyes and slowly run your dominant hand up and down the other arm without making skin contact. Keep your hand approximately two-to-three inches away. Do this until you become sensitive to the heat energy. Notice if you can tell the ever-so-slight temperature difference between your skin and the jewelry you're wearing. Also, notice if you can feel the difference in heat temperature between the more muscular and bony areas. The time it takes to become efficient is directly proportional to the focus and sensitivity you choose to put into this playful practice. This seemingly small exercise will open the doorway to a greater understanding of your human body.

<u>Being Responsible for Your Immune System</u>

Allow this handbook to empower you and its readers to be fully responsible for your health and well-being. It is easy to comprehend, however, accepting responsibility for creating your dis-ease, is another story because it is not something the average person wants to tackle or even admit.

With so much yet to learn about health and dis-ease, the information in this handbook hopes to upgrade your awareness and help survivors thrive inside of a *new normal* lifestyle. Reading and embracing the information in this handbook will help to permanently expand your perspectives on how a healthy mind functions. The options to create a healthier life are now in your hands. Understanding some basic things about the human body may help dispel some of your fears.

<u>Cancer Cells in a Healthy Body</u>[5]

It is vitally essential to understand that every healthy man, woman, and child has millions of cancer cells in their body. Cancer cells are part of cell production in healthy human biology. Like any factory that produces products on an assembly line where quality controllers remove imperfect products, cancer cells also result from the body's mutant cell production. These imperfect cells are a small part of our body's manufacturing system, and our body does its best to treat cancer cells like trash that needs to be periodically taken out to the dumpster.

The primary thing to understand is the importance of the immune system. Your body's immune system is your safeguard for health against most dis-ease. Every effort to regain and maintain your health is directly related to rebuilding the immune system that you continue to unconsciously compromise. Learning how to rebuild your immune system and gain a better opportunity for healthier living is now your lifetime focus. This is not a booby prize but rather a wake-up call to commandeer the quality of your life.

Your body's immune system is designed to create homeostasis and maintain a healthy body. It does its best to minimize cancer cells, keep them at bay, and prevent them from growing into the billions. Like Mother Nature, the body will always find a way to restore and regenerate itself. From bruises to broken bones, your immune system remains committed to a lifetime of healing and works diligently to keep your body thriving until you leave it. It's your job to no longer abuse and disrespect it.

Mistreating your body opens the door to modern medicine being able to see and diagnose a tumor formation and get positive readings from white blood cell counts indicating that cancer cells are growing.

The rule of thumb is that a healthy and balanced body will thrive, and a body fraught with challenges will eventually fail. This is usually due to the mind's belief. When the mind thinks positive and happy thoughts, the body vibrates in good health, and when challenged with negative, unhappy, or fearful thoughts, it causes dis-ease in the body. The body's response tends to be directly proportional to our thoughts.

Our immune system is one of our most incredible lines of defense against disease and is vital for the body to be in great working order. Therefore, it is time to roll up your sleeves and get excited about being fully accountable for it.

A vital perspective shift to have and welcome is being the pilot in your protocol or health management for the rest of your life and giving up your co-pilot's seat. From this moment forward, you may choose many co-pilots to work with. Placing yourself in the driver's seat is a big responsibility and is the most important gift you will ever give to yourself. Once you become the pilot, no one else but you will have the final say on what you do to your body, (aka *earth suit*).

Being 100% responsible and accountable for your life is key to generating a better quality of life for yourself. So before moving forward, let's understand what you've done to get to this point.

Being unaware and desensitized to your immune system was like giving a clinched five-finger fist punch right in the gut.

<u>The Five Finger Punch</u>[6]

1. Poor Diet & Nutrition – Not all food is nutritious. It is probably safe to say that most of your current diet includes processed food and an abundance of sugar on which cancer thrives. A rule of thumb to be aware of is that ingredients that are difficult to pronounce or understand are immediately unwelcome into your body, so be sure to read the packaging labels. Even many sugar-free products are packed with toxic sweetening chemicals. You may find this quite difficult to do all at once, so don't feel bad about revamping your entire food pantry multiple times. Instead, get excited about all your efforts to profoundly alter your life.

2. Lack of Exercise – Compare your sedentary lifestyle and lack of movement to a stagnant pond that eventually develops bacteria, moss, and toxicity. Moderate exercise, without exception, must become your new normal to maintain a healthy mind and body. This is not the time to moan or bitch about it. As Nike says, "Just Do It!"

    How active we remain ultimately determines the overall extent of how good we feel about ourselves. Couch potatoes are not in this category; if you're one of them, you need to recommit to a daily exercise regime instead of grabbing another beer or sweetened soft drink from the refrigerator during television commercials. You can begin with walking and gradually work up to brisk walking.

    Walking is a great activity that keeps your body systems and fluids in motion. Yoga, gym exercise, and any physical activity which are essential for strength and flexibility must be added to a committed degree your new schedule.

3. Lack of Sleep – Adequate sleep helps heal and regenerate all systems in the body, while poor sleep prevents the body from reenergizing itself to take on a new day. Finding ways to gain a deep sleep is now on your list of priorities.

    Night-time showering is a great way to say goodbye to all the negative, yucky 'stuff' that accumulates from the day and helps prepare yourself for a good night's sleep. When you have trouble sleeping, choose from many safe and healthy alternative options online that help you easily feel drowsy. Should you prefer a morning shower to wake you up and feel refreshed, consider throwing water on your face or continuing with your morning shower but still add that nice warm or hot shower at night to wash away the unwanted energies of the day. (Note: Use natural moisturizing oils if your skin becomes too dry)

4. Meditation or Prayer – Not giving yourself time to meditate or pray is neglecting the essential quiet time for your mind to clear from the day's challenges and compromises its flow to generate new thoughts. Quieting down your body and setting good daily intentions, either for yourself or someone you love or care about, leads to internal balance.

5. Stress – You've allowed yourself to be stressed out, and this is your greatest, 'No Pass'! Stress is the worst contributing finger in your fist punch. Your body can only endure a certain amount of stress before it begins to fail and completely break down. Although many of us feel that we can endure anything, stress is not only a considerable booster for all dis-ease, but also scientifically proven to shut the body down and is literally a killer. Simply put, stress suppresses the efficiency of the immune system. This is why, when moving forward, it is imperative to be mindful of what life situations you agree to engage in. Your body is not made of steel and it's nowhere near as resilient as the fictitious characters on television; you must keep in mind they are actors and frequently use their stunt doubles to alleviate their stress.

Those five fingers, which have unconsciously been used to form a hard fist punch to the gut of your immune system, must never happen again!

III. Understanding Cancer Protocols

<u>Understanding Chemotherapy and Radiation</u>[7]

CHEMOTHERAPY:

Although it is an FDA-approved cancer protocol, using chemotherapy is an acceptable poisoning process that comes in different strengths and amounts. The medical industry has been able to prescribe different methods of chemotherapy for different forms of cancer. Having tested it on lab rats and experimented on humans, the American Medical Association (AMA) has allowed various doses as cancer protocols, sometimes resulting in long-term effects on patients. This stems from statistically notating many years of unfavorable results, one of which, is death.

Although advancements have been made, chemotherapy remains a toxic choice designed to kill cancer. There has yet to be any science that prevents chemotherapy from destroying healthy cells simultaneously.

A challenge that cancer patients face is to maintain their weight and build their immune system beforehand, to weather the storm of treatment protocols more successfully. One downside to chemotherapy is that attempts to build the immune system during treatment tend to slow down the effect of chemo and are often frowned upon.

Note: chemotherapy may effectively kill cancer and, at the same time, is known to also cause cancer.

RADIATION:

Radiation is a completely different treatment designed to kill human cells. Unlike chemotherapy, all radiation is always permanent and continues to exist in the body long after the protocol is completed. Post-radiation side effects, such as fibrosis, continue to cause health challenges for the rest of your life. This is why it is the 'gift that keeps on giving.' This quote is often a pathetic attempt to joke about what follows one's protocol. Should you live past your life expectancy, doctor's visits will end, and you will no longer be studied for research data (this is roughly 6-8 years after being considered 'cured'). Rest assured that new symptoms from radiation will appear and how healthy a lifestyle you choose will determine how severe those challenges will be.

Depending on what year you develop cancer will reflect the revised and updated protocols that are/were available. Years ago, radiation levels were administered at levels of 7000 rads. Gradually, the intensity of radioactive waves was reduced; today, it is at 3000 rads. In addition, two decades ago, few attempts were made to suggest or even add aftercare, such as physical therapy, or educate patients on the importance of cleaning up their diets to live a healthier lifestyle. We have certainly come a long way and still have far to go. The day that the AMA finds ways to generate massive income with new licensed and protected healthier ways to cure cancer, chemotherapy, and radiation will come to an end. Until then, this is all they've got to offer, and patients continue to pay dearly in many ways.

Whether the protocol was chemotherapy and/or radiation, foods with high sugar content have been the patient's suggested options to keep their weight up. If you happen to be old enough, you'll remember on television that doctors also preferred people smoking Camel cigarettes over all the other brands. Sharing this is not intended to be disrespectful to the medical profession but rather to speak of their ignorance at the time and underscore that they are human and will prescribe what they are taught and what generates income, directly and indirectly. It is always suggested to show them their due respect and at the same time, lose the God-like worship.

For patients who experienced getting a PT or PET Scan, you may recall being injected with a solution beforehand and resting for an hour. Radioactive sugar isotopes are put into your bloodstream, and the resting time allows the sugar molecules to travel to the cancer sites in your body. This allowed the scan to light up the "hot spots" where the cancer is located. PET scans also tell you when you are cancer-free. This medical protocol illustrates that sugar is like 'filet mignon' to cancer cells and is something you want to remove from your regular diet until your immune system is built back up to the point where it wards off cancer production. Remember, it's normal for our body to produce cancer cells; we rely on our immune system to destroy them.

When you deprive your immune system of good nutrition, don't exercise, have stress, get poor sleep, and do not take the time to calm your mind with prayer or meditation, you compromise and weaken your immune system, preventing it from sufficiently fighting off cancer cells. This ignorance abandons your front line of defense. If you still choose not to shift what's needed to thrive after you learn this information, then you're just being resigned or stupid because you're no longer ignorant. If your mind and body are not past the point of no return, feeding your immune system with high-test nutrition is your best option to maximize your chances of enjoying a healthy life.

Post-Care for Chemotherapy and Radiation

Again, the best post-care for chemotherapy is to do your best to reverse the above – eat healthy, exercise, get deep sleep, achieve effective stress management, and calm your mind daily with prayer or meditation. If you shortchange yourself with this, you increase your chances of relapse because you've not become responsible for that which caused it.

Many folks in America remain clueless about what causes most cancers. We have the highest rate of cancer in the world, and it's not because we are special; we're just ignorant of what living a healthy lifestyle is about and have been a nation of fast and processed foods for decades. Your compromised immune system is the most important consideration, and that's not to say that other outside variables don't encourage the creation of cancer cells. However, it's important to focus on the main contributor to cancer, which is you. Remember, when you compromise your body and weaken your immune system's energetics, dis-ease will impact the weakened energy centers in your body.

Lack of awareness illustrates ignorance; when we are ignorant, we cannot be held accountable. Knowledge and awareness allow for positive action to occur, and for you to be the final decision-maker of your life. It remains in your hands.

Radiation, however, is a horse of a different color. Unlike after chemotherapy, the body fights to return its tissue to a healthier state. Radiated tissue is permanently damaged and continues to migrate throughout the body. Radiation fibrosis is an unwelcome 'gift'; knowing more about its characteristics is imperative to living a 'new normal' life.

Radioactive fibrotic tissue is a new type of tissue. It is brand new to the body and appears after radiation therapy. It, therefore, needs to be treated differently. Until new miracles are understood scientifically, there will not be any valid data or protocol to fully heal these frequently occurring, potentially dangerous, side effects.

Using your common sense and self-assessment are important. Your health and well-being are important. To better understand how fibrotic tissue responds, consider a brand-new rubber band. It's like healthy tissue. It's soft and pliable; when you expand it, it stretches, and you can feel its strength. Fibrotic tissue, on the other hand, is like shoe leather or thin layered like that of a drum. It has little to no moisture and has compromised elasticity. As fibrotic tissue advances, it becomes more obvious to the naked eye.

For your most excellent chances of having the best long-term results with freshly radiated tissue, an immediate protocol following radiation needs to be followed. Patients who are unaware of this will miss out on the advantage of physical therapies to keep their tissue from shrinking or becoming chronically fibrotic. Advanced fibrosis can be life-threatening. Until science knows how to stop the continual spread of radioactive fibrosis, a lifetime of healthy maintenance is needed, and it is completely up to you.

Fibrotic tissue is burned tissue with minimal to no elasticity. A scab that covers a cut or scrape is a perfect example of how the body heals with fibers. However, when fibrotic tissue is beneath the skin, it is also dry. However, the ability for fibrotic tissue to retract can be more painful than when trying to stretch it. Left unattended, fibrotic tissue will continue to shrink to the point of permanently compromising movement and functionality and could compromise the quality of your life in more ways than initially realized.

Treating internal fibrotic tissue can be approached with nutritional supplementation which can help to break up the tissue itself, while external fibrotic tissue is better approached through intentional stretching. Knowing how to stretch fibrotic tissue is very important. In doing so, it's also important to know that fibrotic tissue responds differently than healthy tissue. Stretching this type of tissue for short-term intervals provides only a temporary fix for a better range of motion and suppleness to touch. Therapeutic treatment, however, requires long-held, timed-out stretches to teach this type of tissue to remain more flexible. This is not something that occurs overnight but requires a long-committed effort.

Red Light Therapy (RLT) is a new alternative to healing the body from protocol side effects and helps with external scarring. It is still in its infancy stage yet deserves more delving into the research being done. It appears safe and, unlike Ultraviolet light, may be an option to help alleviate internal fibrotic tissue.

Another new alternative possibility is adding hydrogen-rich water to your daily diet, best taken on an empty stomach. The research is in its infancy, yet the benefits are positive, especially around fibrotic tissue and complete health.

The key approach to take on fibrotic tissue is to adopt an attitude of defiance, blended with a little piss and vinegar for some flair, and commit yourself to an intentional routine of exercise and stretching, along with qualified support from a physical therapist (PT). To date, this is what's available and can be effective.

Some other alternative attempts to return the body to better health and well-being are ozone therapy, stem cell therapy, barometric chambers, and other naturopathic and alternative forms of healing. It is strongly suggested to continually throw out your net and see what you find and feels right for you. If it works, keep it; if not, let it go, and you'll have your own valuable story to tell.

<u>Medical Knowledge and Understanding</u>

From the beginning of mankind, we have looked at ourselves and studied ways to cure illness. In hindsight, many treatments have been unkind and even viewed as prehistoric. Likewise, today's current methods will one day become old and appear as unkind as past protocols, when new practices are implemented. Characteristically we somehow get amnesia when it comes to remaining responsible for learning what we can to sustain the quality of our lives. A conscious practice can only help create the best outcomes for the only human existence we have come to know so intimately.

As a patient searching for professional care, have a 'buyer beware' perspective. Make sure to get a second and even a third opinion to learn as many perspectives as possible before choosing the one that is right for you. Treatment protocols result from great research yet are never set in stone. Learning how your cancer type behaves and metastasizes in general is never exact… because everyone's body is different.

IV. Preparing for a Transformational Reality to Occur

<u>A New Lifestyle to Create and Live Into</u>

Just be open. This not only means learning but also unlearning. Unlearning is vital to one's growth and development. However, the irony is that many of us don't do this effectively, which is why many bad habits remain and the main reason people get 'stuck' in their lives.

Look at your life for a moment, then take time to write down three things that, if you unlearned them, would possibly have something new that works better in your life. Consciously commit to making it a daily practice to do just that and see what is soon to follow.

THINGS I CHOOSE TO UNLEARN

1. ____

2. ____

3. ____

<u>De-Mystifying Cancer and Embracing the Fears Around It</u>

Everyone has cancer cells, and the degree to which they pose a problem is directly proportional to how we manage our bodies. Cancer is only a symptom of the cause. Tumors and lymph nodes are two of the body's miraculous ways of keeping cancer cells contained and protecting them from metastasizing to other parts of the body. Once they are discovered and before a medical protocol is established, it is imperative for the patient to come to an immediate stop and reevaluate their nutrition and lifestyle. This requires a complete mind reset and focused effort. Knowledge is power, and it is the road less traveled at this crossroad. Being fully responsible and accountable for the quality of your life is not easy because nothing worthwhile ever is. However, you are worth it! The primary focus at this point should be to do what is essential to rebuilding the body's immune system immediately (organic nutrition, exercise, adequate sleep, meditation/prayer, and the removal of all stress from your life). Knowing this could prevent the biggest mistake most of us make, which is not to create a stronger immune system immediately after diagnosis. Altering diet and lifestyle can help shrink and remove encapsulated cancerous tumors and lymph nodes from the body without cancer protocols and/or reduce the severity of treatment. The protocol that doctors recommend at this point is to do a needle biopsy or removal of a piece of tumor for testing purposes.

Sadly, these two processes leak cancer cells into the body, increasing the chances of cancer spreading should it go untreated. If you are afraid now, it needs to be replaced with awareness and alertness for doing what is needed to better govern your body and minister to building the healthiest immune system as quickly as possible. Oxygen and alkalinity are key to a healthy body because they support your immune system by creating an environment for cancer cells to lose their vitality and die.

Short-Circuiting Cancer From Existing or Returning – The BIG Secret About Cancer Prevention

Plain and straightforward, cancer cannot live in an alkaline and oxygenated environment. That's it! Cancer loves acidity, sugar (which is highly acidic), and less oxygenated places in the body, to grow and develop.

When a person is diagnosed with cancer of any kind and if time is not of the essence to treat it, a three-month regime of organic alkaline nutrition and oxygenation under professional supervision would be ideal to return the body to health or reduce the severity of cancer. This may be something to consult a naturopathic physician or qualified health professional. Keep in mind that there are places where people who were considered terminally ill have gone for treatment and left weeks later cancer-free.[8]

What the body needs most for either a cure or a remission, is to immediately switch to a healthy high-alkaline diet, removing all sugar, increasing water intake to more than half your body weight in ounces, and giving it plenty of oxygen, such as fresh air walks, hyperbaric chamber sessions, or ozone therapy treatments.

Once again, every healthy body has millions of cancer cells that the immune system helps to remove. However, when you are grossly overweight (30 pounds or more by national standards) or morbidly obese (80-188 pounds or more), you've loaded your body with sugar and simple carbohydrates that instantly break down into sugar, too. Sugar is the precursor to many diseases that Americans face. How many people do you know with cancer, diabetes, stroke, and all the illnesses associated with obesity? Almost 60% of our nation's population is overweight, and it's a result of the toxicity generated from fast and processed foods and lack of exercise. This is also information you'll want to take to heart now.

The task at hand is to realize that your nutrition and lifestyle have created the disease in your body and that only a 180° turn around will be what it takes to say goodbye to cancer without the possibility of recurrence. This is a bold perspective and one that can work effectively.

<u>Knowledge is Self-Empowerment</u>

Although fear is a great motivator, self-empowerment is an even greater one. Realizing that you are the key source of your dis-ease is initially unsettling and simply doesn't feel good. However, realizing that you are also the source of your wellness, is an amazing opportunity for you to run the show regarding how things go for the rest of your life. So often, we give our power away and find ourselves at the effect of a situation. Taking permanent ownership is the key to empowering life's experiences because you can hold onto your core center and maintain the free will to choose what is right for you. Knowing that you are your ship's captain allows you to be the one who charts the course. This is your opportunity to finally wake up to your power center and take ownership for the remainder of your lifetime. At that moment, the medical or other professionals you trust become your co-pilots and will willingly serve you. From their perspective, a patient who shows great initiative makes their job easier. Take charge, know your alternatives, and stand for the level of service you deserve. You are the pilot of your journey.

V. Healthier Living

<u>The Great Challenge and Shift That Is Needed</u>

Turning your life around health-wise requires you to look at all the processed foods[9] you consume. Most of them are considered food, but not all "nutrition". A question to ask yourself is, "What will feed and create cancer, a can of Coke and some Pringles or Water and some Roasted Organic Vegetables?" Not all answers will be this obvious, and after you become aware, the next hurdle to get over is the challenge of unlearning bad habits.

We can go on and on with the obvious, but you've got the point. Start to read all labels on packaged and processed foods you currently have in your cupboards and immediately pitch everything with ingredients you can't pronounce.

As a side note, did you know that pouring Coca-Cola on a car removes the paint? Coke is also a home remedy for rust removal.[10] A car is made of metal, so think of what it does to the soft, supple live tissue in your digestive tract. Please ponder the possible impact that tissue deterioration will eventually have from consuming carbonated sugared drinks.

A frightening statistic to realize is that if the entire planet understood the healing ramifications of healthy nutrition and decided to all eat organically to live a cleaner lifestyle, there would not be enough produced to sustain everyone.

The continued formula to grow populations of unhealthy people required learning to consume processed foods. Anything manufactured and presented in a box, a can, or a bag has a good possibility of being processed food with unnatural additives that are offensive to the human body. It's not your body's friend unless it comes from the earth, void of pesticides and other pollutants. Consuming animals treated with antibiotics and growth hormones and eating foods sprayed with pesticides is a subject for another time.

The overall process of waking up to cleaner living is best likened to peeling layers of an onion. To unlearn what you've learned all these years and learn new ways of living takes focused intention and follow-through with action. Human nature has proven that folks who gladly take on a challenge such as this, are the ones who have had a life-threatening illness and choose to be responsible for it to never happen again. People who are 'fat and happy', as it is coined, are more likely to be stuck inside their routine lives and unwilling to make changes due to complete laziness.

The Mind's Thoughts are Directly Proportional to the Body's Physical Response

Although it may not be seen or felt right away, thoughts immediately affect the body and can eventually impact its physiology.

The longer you stay awake, the easier it is to sense the physiological shifts. Although not all body parts are easy to sense, you can begin by focusing on your gut. The gut, which is often thought to be solely in your stomach, happens to be the entire digestive system from your mouth to your anus and the end of your urinary tract. When asked to 'trust their gut', the information is derived from that entire system and felt mainly in the tummy.

As we learn to become more sensitive to our *earth suit*, we notice more nuances which we eventually grow to trust as reliable. However, in the beginning, like with any practice, we tend to miss quite a bit and realize these shifts later. For instance, if you binge on sweets and carbohydrates, although the energetic shift can occur within minutes, it may take hours before you don't feel well and won't have any confirmation until the next day when you step onto the scale or possibly have diarrhea. As you sensitize and focus on any physiological energy shifts in the body, you'll begin to feel the subtle signs of impact without needing to wait until later.

The Practice of Unlearning and Reprogramming a New Thought System

This, for certain, is a life-long commitment, and who better than you to commit yourself to for your lifetime?

The well-known saying, "To think, therefore I am," is a nice tidbit of wisdom; however, it may be more poignant if combined with "and to re-think, therefore I become," as an attachment. This will allow expansive thinking to occur more frequently and abundantly.

Your sense of self-worth and internal power increases when you allow yourself to unlearn bad habits and substitute them with good ones.

Stop and pause briefly and write down five things worth learning more about. Think of anything associated with that task that may require unlearning before you begin. This will help make you better equipped when deciding what to put into your body and how you intend to navigate throughout life.

THINGS WORTH LEARNING MORE ABOUT

1.____

2.____

3.____

4.____

5.____

A New Way to Exercise - Put Fun, Play, and Exuberance Into It!

Why haven't we made exercise fun? Some people seem to have a highly allergic reaction to it! This is so uncool and what many of us need to unlearn and reprogram our minds with a new perspective of joy, fun, and ease. This requires delving into. Take some time to explore.

Creative ways to have fun exercising are to enroll others into exercising with you or ask what they do to accomplish their daily exercise. Let's unlearn the 'misery loves company' belief and create new thoughts that will allow you to exceed your expectations. The time is now to create and implement this. Somehow, somewhere, you've agreed to see exercise as drudgery. Now it's time to imprint a new and more appropriate perspective on your mind.

A Lifestyle Shift in Nutrition – Not All Food is Nutrition[11]

First, it might be a good idea to become more aware of the foods you enjoy, liquids included. Make a bulleted list of all the foods and beverages you consume monthly. Make sure you do a complete brain dump of this. Next to each one, enter how often you consume them. Notice any patterns and remember that too much of anything is not good. The key is balance!

FOODS AND BEVERAGES I CONSUME EACH MONTH AND HOW OFTEN						

After you're done, highlight the items that are the most toxic, and cut and paste them into a list of foods you'll want to avoid.

NEVER TO EAT AGAIN FOODS			

Next, make a list of less toxic foods that you choose to eat in moderation.

Foods to Eat in Moderation			

After you've created these three lists, make a fourth list of foods that you know are the best kinds of foods to eat, and add the types of foods you don't like but know are good for you.

Nutrition I Choose to Eat For the Rest of My Life			

Place the food items you can't stand at the bottom of the page until you're open to incorporating them into your diet. This will help you feel better about the list.

When you begin to peel away the layers of your toxic foods from your diet and begin to add in the nutrition that your body so desperately craves as a higher-test fuel, at that time, you may consider adding foods you never thought possible that would be allowed into your body. Have fun with this and add some excitement because you are making this a pivotal moment where significant shifts are about to occur.

How My Body Reacts to Sugar[12]

Think of "erosion" and "decay," and you'll get an instant picture. There are way too many obvious health challenges that arise from sugar consumption, especially processed sugar and sugar substitutes. You're welcome to research this but rest assured, processed sugar and substitutes are foreign and toxic to your body.

Recalling that if you had a PET Scan during your cancer treatment, radioactive sugar isotopes were injected into your body. You were asked to lie still for 30-45 minutes, allowing the radioactive isotopes to migrate directly to the cancer sites, wherever they might be. This allows the scan to light up these "Hot Spots" areas.

The reason is because sugar is like filet mignon to cancer. Sugar helps cancer grow and metastasize to other areas of the body.

A healthy body with significant amounts of sugar surely has a predictable fate.

<u>Flexibility is KEY</u>

Flexibility pertains to your mind, body, and spirit… spirit being the most flexible of the three. Then comes the mind, followed by the body.

As we age, many people pride themselves on having a lucid mind and clear thinking. The aging process doesn't guarantee this to everyone. Therefore, not only is it a gift but something that requires effort from you to achieve. Remember that recreational as well as some prescription drugs, in addition to alcohol, are significant factors that compromise lucid brain function, so be mindful of the side effects.

Finally, the body. Unless you've been a gymnast or athlete from childhood and have been highly active throughout your adult life, an average body stiffens and shrinks over time, becoming inflexible, arthritic, and hunched over. Healthy bodies maintain the same height, weight, and stature, while average bodies do not.

<u>The ULTIMATE Lifestyle</u>

The Ultimate Diet – Live organic produce[13] and wild fish caught in uncontaminated waters. Many folks resist this because they feel it's way too expensive. Granted, it's a bit more. However, you must fill it with high-grade, clean nutrition to create a healthy body. It's time to realize that affordability is prioritized over limited finance. As you create your nutritional palate of foods, think of it this way: If it's from the earth and comes out of salt or fresh water to the table, it's probably good for you. In addition, the only liquid for the Ultimate Diet is clean mountain water and sometimes distilled water. A minimum daily consumption amount to keep your body hydrated is half your body weight in ounces. Distilled water is considered 'hungry water' because of its ability to attract unwanted particles throughout the body, and it is ideal when it's time for a detoxification cleansing.

The Ultimate Physical Activity – To repeat what we already know; thirty to sixty minutes of brisk walking is a great way to enjoy a new sunrise. The morning is the best time to soak in the sun's rays because they are the lowest in ultraviolet rays and, as consistently, high in vitamin D. It's important to include stretching. Therefore, consider learning yoga because it allows you to stretch fully. Yoga, plus a moderate workout with weights, will help bless you with a great night's sleep. Sleep is critical in helping your body regenerate, revitalize, and refresh. Granted, the ultimate lifestyle almost seems unattainable, so take it step by step, enjoy what you can do, and keep aspiring for a greater expression of yourself.

Again, make this fun and something to begin tomorrow, or aspire to start soon. If you're already active or are doing one or two of these, it's time to add another until you're fully up and running.

The Ultimate Mindset – The repetition here is solely for purposes of reinforcement. Meditation and prayer are essential in giving your mind a well-needed colonic (brain enema). With approximately 65,000 thoughts going through your mind daily, it gets crowded inside. A warm-to-hot shower helps eliminate the day's negative energy in your body. Meditation helps to flush away the day's challenges and is an outlet for stress relief. Adding prayers after your meditation can help to set some positive and powerful intentions for a new day.

VI. A Day in the Life of a Thriving Cancer Survivor

<u>Waking up to Meditation and Setting Your Intentions for the Day</u>

Upon waking each morning, wipe the sleep out of your eyes, splash your face with soothing warm water, and empty your bladder. This is the perfect time to set a timer for 30-45 minutes and allow your mind to cleanse itself by thinking of nothing but your breathing. Thoughtlessness[14] is the goal but not a deal breaker if you are a beginner. What's important is that your mind is clearer each time you are done. After your meditation, reset the timer for 10-15 minutes and place a strong focus on creating intentions of how you'd like to see your day unfold. This allows you to create a day of your own design. Picture your day going as planned, then be mindful of what you had intended throughout the day. This is your creation, and you are running the show. Stay aware, be responsible for your thinking, and have fun making it happen. Be sure not to hold onto any expectations of outcome. You may not see your visions turn out exactly the way you intended. Rather, they may have far exceeded your expectations if you allow surprises and serendipity to occur.

<u>What's in Your Kitchen Cabinets and Pantry? – Suggested Food Supplements</u>

Take the opportunity to open all your cabinets and take pictures with your cell phone of what's inside. Do this with your refrigerator, too. You will be unpleasantly surprised! It's time to purge the foods that create physical dis-ease and hold onto whatever good nutrition is left.

These are your enlightenment photos and your wake-up call to action. A new day has begun in the life of a transformed cancer survivor!

Choosing the right foods is as easy as ABC. Anything that's not organic, processed with ingredients you're unfamiliar with, or can't pronounce easily must go.

Supplements are easily found at a health food market. Asking for help from a vitamin and supplement associate makes life much easier. They are surprisingly knowledgeable regarding whatever supplement you need for what ails you or what you are trying to achieve. It's even easier to research any ailment you may have online and learn about its natural remedy. There are seemingly endless websites selling products you can have shipped right to your door. This is service at its best. Keep in mind that not all vitamins and supplements are created equal. The greatest differences are in both the product quality and their absorption rate, therefore buyer beware.

<u>Vitamins, Minerals, and Things to Add to Your Meals</u>

It is important to search for supplements that boost your immune system, improve each organ's health, and increase muscle mass. After having a routine blood test to determine what your body is deficient in, you can choose healthier options over medication. There is a need and purpose for medication, but choosing a natural route needs to become your preference. Remember, with the proper nutrition and supplements, your body should continue healing. If you take a medication, count on side effects with no contribution to helping your body produce what it needs to return to health on its own. Be mindful of those side effects!

When beginning a new routine of vitamins and minerals for the body's health, it is important to read the recommended daily allowance (RDA) on each package, then consider multiplying the dosage by two, three, or four, depending on the product and what you'd like to achieve. The RDA is often for healthy maintenance guidelines and is oftentimes insufficient to achieve a noticeable difference. After taking the increased dose for three to four weeks, see if you feel a difference. If you feel a difference, lower the dose by one for another two to three weeks, after which you can either lower it again or follow the recommended amount. You get to choose. Note: If you're familiar with muscle testing, that may be a good guide to help select dosage.

Instead of taking all your supplements in the morning, consider incorporating them into shakes and titrating them into your system throughout your day. Some supplements will tell you if they are more effective on an empty stomach. Getting maximum benefit from your supplements is key.

<u>Immune System and Fighting the Common Cold</u>

With all that is known in naturopathic medicine, you no longer need to take the common cold lying down. High doses of Vitamin C, intravenously or orally, can be taken in large quantities throughout the day.[15] If your GI tract can handle it, consider that 20k – 30k milligrams of Vitamin C will end a cold within two to three days. There are no contraindications to overdosing on the Internet, and it is always recommended that you check with your medical team before attempting this. Use the Internet to research because this is uncharted territory in modern medicine.

Note: Lower the dosage if Vitamin C upsets your stomach or gives you loose bowels. Also note that it's important to know that although a cold virus is common, some strains can destroy the cochlea in the ear and render an individual completely deaf. Being grateful for your life, which is temporary, and being mindful of a common cold is being responsible.

<u>Nutrition for Champions, Intermittent Fasting, and Fasting</u>

Organic nutrition is the best fuel for optimizing great health, like breathing in clean air, drinking pure water, and consuming two to three meals daily. When you are inspired to "up your game", this will be another layer of the onion you've peeled to reach the next level of purer nutrition of what your body needs to thrive.

Another special gift for your body is intermittent fasting,[16] where you choose a span of four to six hours in your day, and with water being the only exception, use that time to consume your daily nutrition. This gives your body ample downtime to assimilate what you've put into it. Intermittent fasting has been around for many years and has great advantages to keep your digestive system in great working order. Eating three square meals daily (morning, afternoon, and evening), is old-school thinking. However, should you still enjoy three meals throughout your day, consider having a moderate healthy breakfast to give your body the fuel it needs to start your day. Follow with your largest meal at lunchtime, when your body has plenty of time to easily digest it. You may enjoy a fresh fruit snack around 3 pm - 4 pm if you need a natural energy boost. Contrary to popular tendencies, dinner should be your smallest meal – keep it light. Depending on your dinner time, it can remain stuck in your gut for most of the night. A good rule of thumb is not to have anything to eat or drink three hours before sleep.

Another school of thought, especially concerning losing weight, is to eat small portions steadily throughout the day. Doing so keeps your body constantly digesting without the rest it needs for other bodily functions and regenerating itself. This type of eating should be temporary (up to seven days at a time). Be sure to check with your nutritionist or doctor before taking this route. This purpose is to awaken a sleepy digestive tract and is not for optimum health.

Note: If you reference animals in the wild, the ones that eat only when they find their prey, they are usually leaner and more fit. The animals that graze all day tend to be healthy, too, but a bit more filled out.

VII. Placing the Medical World in Proper Perspective - Getting Real

For the past decade or so, after all the tobacco companies were banned from national television airways, the pharmaceutical companies dedicated themselves to having a huge influence on national TV advertising. Ever since then, they have been in their glory. With all their commercials so brilliantly constructed, they sell their drugs directly to you, their consumer. The repetition and abundance of commercials is a proven formula to make you believe that taking their drugs will help you. The commercials are also intended to desensitize you to the point of overlooking all the adverse side effects of the medication. Most patient's next step is to ask their doctor for a prescription. Doctors, without disrespect, have become glorified order takers for 'big pharma.'[17] Doctors have gone from once being revered as all-knowing gods to glorified prescription writers.

In addition to surgeries and other procedures, doctors have studied very diligently in medical school to have a license to practice pharmaceutical medicine on humans. It is also important to understand that pharmaceutical companies help medical schools in many ways, including financially. This is not by accident. Although there is a very strong bonded relationship with big pharma, all doctors take the oath to help care for the sick and do no harm. Gradually, there has been more effort made within the medical industry to incorporate wellness considerations instead of just managing the patient by only removing the symptoms. There remains, however, little interest in addressing the causes of dis-ease.

Although there aren't any hard facts about it, common sense would tell us that if most people were educated on disease causes, the need for many medical providers would diminish. Large corporations and manufacturers hire professionals determined by supply and demand for many products and services.

People are people, and doctors are people, too. They come in all shapes and sizes, temperaments, and levels of intelligence. An old joke once told was, "What's the difference between a doctor and a god?" The answer: "A doctor knows they're a doctor!" Those referenced doctors have huge egos, and patients treat them like gods. However, this is not the case for most newer patients and medical professionals. Doctors are here to serve their patients in the best manner they know. The major irony is that medical school is the factory they've been put through and is inundated with pharmaceutical influence. In addition, med-students have not been taught to gain understanding from a whole-body educational approach. They are slowly getting there because their patients are more well-educated and inquisitive. Doctors now have the opportunity to attend alternative medical seminars, which can be applied to their continued educational credit requirement.

However, most doctors are swamped with patients and have overloaded schedules, making attending challenging.

The takeaway here is to place your medical support team in their proper place and allow them to shift from initial pilots to co-pilots. This provides you with the freedom to consider all options available to you.

<u>Where Do You Stand in the Lineup?</u>

Initially, it is important to interview as many qualified and referred medical professionals as possible when dealing with any illness. Some qualified people might even be PAs and other support staff to the medical doctors. Once you have found the one(s) you like most, learn what they know so that you confirm for yourself that they can best assist you. To give them your reins without understanding them first places you in a dependency position that may come around to haunt you later on.

Knowledge is powerful, and many doctors are pleasantly surprised to see their patients playing an active role in their protocol because it helps reassure them that their patients will be better equipped to live their lives more responsibly with a lower rate of dis-ease reoccurrence. Most doctors enjoy seeing their patients actively working with them and adding information to conversations. If you notice that they are taken back negatively, you'll want to leave skid marks and high-tail them out of their office! Those doctors prefer passive patients who follow their instructions and don't think for themselves.

When spending time with your doctor(s), it's empowering for you to make them aware that they are your co-pilot so that you are more fully present in what is being created for you to soldier through. During your first time meeting them, you may sense a go-ahead to seek out a second opinion and/or alternative ways, like exercise and nutritional programs, that will help boost your results and their statistics. Remember, you are allowing yourself to be their patient. They have a license to 'practice' medicine on you, and all patients, including you, are recorded and charted for medical statistics. This underscores the importance of your role as the pilot of your protocol.

VIII. Miracles Happen Every Day and You Are One of Them!

The sad news is that many people don't make it through the challenging treatments of radiation and chemotherapy, and the good news is that you are still here! The question is, "What will you do with the time you've been given?"

When it's our time to die, we will. No one gets off this planet alive, and those who have had a near-death experience may remember the beyond-words magnificence that awaits after we leave our bodies.

Now is your opportunity to open your heart and mind and be willing to allow more miracles to occur. Miracles occur daily when you're able to see them. Doing this requires focus and sensitivity to the energetics of things that allow a shift in perspective. It's much like taking your sunglasses off and putting on reading glasses that allow you to see more clearly.

The human body is miraculous. Ask anyone who has studied it. Medical science has learned much about it, but they have yet to know it all. There are so many things we are still learning about. The mind, the body's energy vibrations, the intelligence of the gut (the entire system between the mouth and the anus), and the fact that one cell has more intelligence than the entire brain itself are all still mysteries to us as we continue to discover more about them. Remember, miracles are nothing more than unknown facts. Once we discover what makes a miracle a miracle, it's no longer a miracle but a scientific reality. But also remember, scientific facts are never true because they are clearer perceptions that often change over time.

At one time, science used visual acuity to confirm that the world was flat and that the sun revolved around the Earth. This underscores that it's best to remain in the inquiry instead of the findings. The findings are real at the time but never true. This is because the truth implies one way only and cannot be changed. Anything that can be altered by a shift in perspective was never true.

No matter how much effort human science makes to continually try to *figure things out,* we always live in an uncertain world. Therefore, it's time to be more responsible and accountable and trust our gut instincts for how we choose to navigate through life.

Consider writing your own handbook. It doesn't need to be published, although it can be. Let it be a handbook that confirms a new way of living that has made the greatest difference for yourself. Imagine sharing a new perspective on life that allows you to thrive.

IX. Your Lifeline - Finding the Team of Experts to Support You

Having the right team of people who will support you will determine the quality of your life. This team of educated professionals will change and morph over time, which is good. Chances are they may not be covered by your insurance, which will require you to prioritize finding a way to maintain their support. New research findings are published daily and take time to show up in public view, so patience and perseverance are key. To authentically hold your support team dear to your heart, you and they must all agree to be respectfully human. This means that everyone respects one another for what they bring to the table. This will guarantee a quality long-term relationship.

<u>A Great Physical Therapist</u>

Your Physical Therapist (PT) will help keep your body flexible as fibrotic tissue infiltrates other areas. Post-radiation fibrotic advancement, coupled with a sedentary lifestyle, will result in your loss of flexibility. To date, radiation does not stop the dirty deed of infiltration. Many patients are not forewarned of this because, other than chemotherapy, it remains a thriving and profitable protocol in modern medicine. Not every PT is alike, and although trained in general studies, they may have their own areas of expertise. Finding out and questioning them ongoingly is vital for clarity's sake.

Suggestion: Look for Physical Therapists with a track record working with cancer patients and fibrotic tissue. Although there are always exceptions, the rule of thumb is if they are fresh out of school, they still haven't learned the information and techniques that you need. If they are too old, they may be missing valuable up-to-date research. Most PTs are upfront and honest, want what's best for you, and will gladly refer you to their colleagues. A PT with 10-15 years of experience is generally needed for this knowledge and hands-on treatment.

<u>A Great Speech and Swallowing Therapist</u>

Unlike all other areas of the body that are treated with radiation, head and neck cancer patients require a speech and swallowing therapist to get them through their post-care. The most important functions that sustain your life occur from the bottom of your neck to the top of your head; eating, swallowing, seeing, hearing, and breathing are critical to living a healthy and sustainable life.

Remember: Be certain that the speech and swallowing therapist has a background in radiation science and how fibrotic tissue impacts the body's functioning.

A Great Dentist, Endodontist, and Oral Surgeon

If your protocol required you to pull all your teeth prophylactically, it's a bit too late if you're reading this now because that was the standard protocol years ago. The higher doses of radiation being administered to the head and neck made for a much higher risk of bone necrosis, which remains a slow death sentence because of the difficulty in treating and healing it.

Radiation often removes the well-needed blood supply to the mouth and compromises your salivary function.

A radiation therapy called IMRT Painting was created years ago to help localize the radiation streams and pinpoint the appropriate cancer targets. This was also created as an attempt to save some salivary function. Patients treated in this manner usually continue to have a portion of their salivary function left intact.

The IMRT protocol was proven to do less damage to surrounding tissue. This helped to slow down the progression side effects that would inevitably make the same appearance as general radiation therapy.

A Great Naturopathic Physician

Unfortunately, health insurance does not cover these professionals because we currently have 'sick care,' not 'health care.' Naturopathic Physicians are well-needed and are an informative addition to standard care. They are innovative and seek to treat the cause and symptoms. Unfortunately, they have been seen as a threat to the AMA's position in the marketplace instead of an ally.

There are multiple things that naturopaths can do that add to recovery. For example, oxygenating the blood with ozone therapy, using vitamin drips to supercharge your immune system, and suggesting stronger and more effective supplements than you may already be taking are only a portion of how they can help to return your body to health.

A Great Exercise Workout Partner

Solo gym workouts are great for the mind to reset itself and feel invigorated. However, if you're not a committed gym rat or don't work out vigorously, having a buddy system might be your answer. It brings fun, excitement, and comradery into the mix and keeps you invigorated and on task in a routine.

Although building muscle mass is important for a healthy body to thrive, it is also important to achieve greater flexibility. As we age, the body becomes less flexible, which is considered normal, but it's not... it's average. What's normal is a healthy body that is honored by being as flexible and limber as can be throughout your life.

Remember: Your miraculous immune system is designed to return your body to how it usually functions. Unfortunately, that is not the current average.

A Great Yoga Studio

Flexibility, stamina, endurance, peace of mind, and more, can be found in yoga. There's no substitute for yoga when it comes to combining the body's flexibility and learning how to gain laser focus on your breath and being present. If you are adventurous, hot yoga is a real treat. Hot yoga helps make it easier and quicker for your body to become flexible. Once you become a yogi by committing to six months to a year of practice, it will surely become part of your new lifestyle.

A Great Nutritionist

This is by far a main event in transforming your physical health. Not all nutritionists are the same, so learn about their school of study (organic or holistic nutritionists are the preferred choice).

Although it is said that you are what you eat, this is not the case at all. Rather, you are what you absorb because not everything you eat is absorbed. More importantly, many foods that are eaten are not always nutritious. The ultimate nutritional lifestyle is to consume all raw organic produce, nuts, seeds, and wild-caught fish minutes to hours after being caught. Unless you live and go fishing near the sea, the average person needs to be more realistic in finding diets that are a hybrid to the ultimate.

If you are committed to never having a recurrence of cancer again, your immune system must be revered as the most important system in your body. This handbook has made a clear attempt to underscore and emphasize the value of your immune system. Chances are it was either ignorance or negligence that got you into trouble in the first place. You must never be like the average person again, but set your sights much higher and be unreasonable. Partnering with a nutritionist, at least at first, will bring greater insight into different food options, food pairing, portion amounts, and eating times. There's so much to explore in the world of nutrition that it can seem overwhelming. Stay the course and have fun with it.

A great nutritionist will begin where you are and slowly and painlessly help you to morph into a diet that is best for you unless you give them the OK to turbo-charge things full steam ahead.

The internet is also a valuable source of information and can be your go-to for more advanced learning regarding nutrition. The nutritionist already has the foundational information you need and will save you a lot of time researching the basics. Remember to use all resources that are available to you.

<u>A Great General Practitioner – Your Primary Co-Pilot</u>

A good General Practitioner (GP) is essential. They are not specialists but the hub of your medical history, and it's best to consider them your home base. Good GPs who balance their medical knowledge with factual alternative care are hard to find because of the country's health care condition. So, you may need to research a few before choosing one that works for you.

Most People agree that the entire healthcare system needs an overhaul. However, until then, find a GP that you love. They can be MD's, DO's, PA's, etc. Also, consider that doctors are as good as their staff, mainly because they hired them. If they are not nice or accommodating, you may have issues. Also, be sure to keep your eyes on their staff. The same rule applies when you get married because you marry family along with all their beliefs and customs. Remember that your spouse grew up in that culture before they became your spouse. Your doctor's staff are their extended family as well.

<u>A Great Hospital</u> (Teaching hospitals preferred)

In the past, many hospitals were not teaching hospitals. Today, it's common for hospitals to supervise interns, although that doesn't make it a teaching hospital. Teaching hospitals educate new professionals on things they may not have learned in medical school. Interns are our future doctors, and although they lack the experience you may need, hopefully, they have learned the latest protocols in medical school.

<u>A Great University</u>

Many larger universities offer their graduate students supervised clinics open to the public, giving them a greater head start before they begin their internship elsewhere.

Patients are comforted by the comradery of a team and tend to have an overall positive experience with this type of health care. Universities often teach the most up-to-date patient treatment protocols and have an inside view of hospitals and doctors. This can be to a person's advantage should they need medical or hospital care.

Again, the culmination of collected resources makes up the quality of support for your lifeline.

X. Finding Support Groups Near You

It's important to know that you are not alone; support groups help you realize that. Having the support of personal friends and family is critical. However, embracing a new community of people who have gone through what you have is essential to not flying solo on your permanently altered life.

Many hospitals offer support groups today. Researching online is a fast and easy way to discover the groups that suit you.

The group leader will often invite experts, clinicians, and other speakers, who will bring you helpful and well-needed research data. You're free to question them to learn what they know and offer your perspective.

Science is constantly changing. For example, the maximum amount of radiation 20+ years ago was 6500 rads of radiation. Eighteen years ago, it dropped to 5000 rads. Today, it's only 3000 rads. This is fortunate for those future patients who are yet to receive their protocol because their predecessors have endured the brutality from which appropriate adjustments were made. Support groups are key in getting the word out, too. Giving keynote speakers your feedback also teaches them about the effects of treatment, which is valuable information for them to take back to the powers that be. It's the same when you meet with your specialists.

Knowing that radiation remains in the body for a lifetime, support groups allow you to see how well other people are progressing after their treatment. Keeping your body as healthy as possible is your best defense.

XI. Unexpected Words of Wisdom

In closing this handbook, here are a few last words to share:

- Whatever options present themselves in any moment that inspires you, choose and own them to the core of your being.

- Act on your choice and take it as far as possible, having the greatest amount of integrity to see it through to completion.

- Make no assumptions nor have any expectations of how you wish things should turn out. Place no claim on how you should make achievements happen and place no expectations on the outcome.

Everything you need to support you will be available during this process.

You are the engine but not the one who's driving. Let universal energy and the laws of synchronicity take that seat.

Allow your mind to open and witness your consciousness expand.

Embrace whatever new perspectives come into view and make them yours.

Whatever you think, feel, and believe is your new reality.

Realities are infinite, so choose your thoughts, feelings, and beliefs wisely, and know that it's everyone's prerogative to alter their reality at a moment's notice.

A great sadness in life is never our death but that which we allow to die inside of us while we are still alive.

I hope and wish that this handbook has provided you with added knowledge and inspiration to be even more responsible for your health and well-being. Remember that you are the captain of your human life-ship, and it is your responsibility to take this opportunity to live the life you're given as intentionally as you can so that when you come to the finish line, you will take your last breath having no regrets, and with a huge smile on your face! (I do my best to remind myself of this every day!)

– Ron Baron

Endnotes

1. Head and neck cancers | Risk factors. (2024). https://www.mayoclinic.org/diseases-conditions/head-and-neck-cancers/symptoms-causes/syc-20354171

2. Head and neck cancers | Treatments. https://www.hopkinsmedicine.org/radiation-oncology/conditions-we-treat/head-neck-cancers#:~:text=External%20beam%20radiation%20is%20the,in%20a%20well%2Ddefined%20region

3. Energetic tendencies (2018). https://www.sciencedirect.com/science/article/pii/S2095754818300358

4. Hay, Louise. You can heal your life (1984). https://www.hayhouse.com/you-can-heal-your-life-paperback

5. Does everyone have cancer cells in their body? (2023). https://www.medicalnewstoday.com/articles/does-everyone-have-cancer-cells-in-their-body

6. Healthy habits: Enhancing immunity (2023). https://www.cdc.gov/healthy-weight-growth/about/enhancing-immunity.html

7. What's the difference between chemotherapy and radiation? (2022). https://www.webmd.com/cancer/cancer-chemotherapy-radiation-differences

8. Clinical review of alkalization therapy in cancer treatment (2022). https://pmc.ncbi.nlm.nih.gov/articles/PMC9516301/

9. How do processed foods affect your health? (2023). https://www.medicalnewstoday.com/articles/318630

10. Did you know Coke could strip away paint? (2017). https://diyeverywhere.com/2017/05/28/did-you-know-coke-could-strip-away-paint-here-are-13-surprising-uses/

11. Nutrition, food and diet in health and longevity: We eat what we are (1922). https://pmc.ncbi.nlm.nih.gov/articles/PMC9785741/

12. The sugar and cancer connection (2016). https://www.aicr.org/news/the-sugar-cancer-connection/

13. Organic foods: Are they safer? More nutritious? (2022). https://www.mayoclinic.org/healthy-lifestyle/nutrition-and-healthy-eating/in-depth/organic-food/art-20043880

14. Mindfulness meditation: A research-proven way to reduce stress (2019). https://www.apa.org/topics/mindfulness/meditation

15. Vitamin C for immunity & disease prevention with Dr. Andrew Saul (2021). https://share.snipd.com/episode/11a62b3c-c546-4f08-8de3-d8bc74a7f79c

16. What is intermittent fasting? Does it have health benefits? (2022),
https://www.mayoclinic.org/healthy-lifestyle/nutrition-and-healthy-
eating/expert-answers/intermittent-fasting/faq-20441303

17. Doctors prescribe more of a drug if they receive money from a
pharma company tied to it (2019).
https://www.propublica.org/article/doctors-prescribe-more-of-a-
drug-if-they-receive-money-from-a-pharma-company-tied-to-it

About the Author

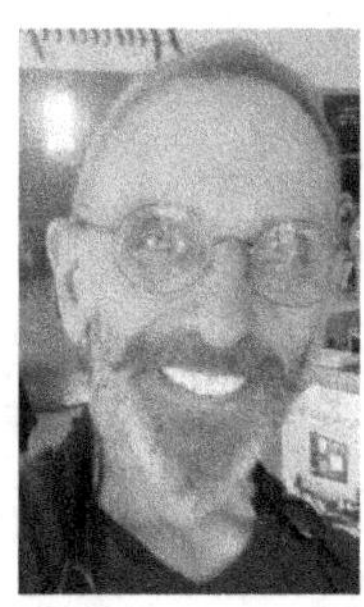

The impetus for writing this handbook was seeing the need to help people become aware of their power center and gain a more comprehensive perspective of what being fully responsible and accountable for their health and well-being looks like. I had a three to six-month-to-live diagnosis of a very rare form of head and neck cancer at the age of 47; it often takes a life-threatening challenge or something significant to stop people in their tracks, redirect their attention from the daily repetitious routines, and refocus on what is more important in life. My diagnosis did just that.

The folks who have gone through the same chemotherapy and radiation protocol as I did in the past either died undergoing their treatment or only lived an additional nine years. As of 2024, I'm currently 18 years cancer-free, and with a defiant spirit, I am still counting. Years have taught me how to prevent cancer from growing uncontrollably inside my body. Surprisingly, modern medicine continues to use the same but modified cancer protocols without knowing how to undo the brutal long-term and life-threatening side effects caused by radiation fibrosis.

With a commitment to clean living, an active lifestyle, healthy nutrition options, and a continual search for alternative approaches to more excellent health and well-being, my journey continues.

For those who seek and lean toward conventional cancer therapies, I strongly suggest doing your homework first. In hindsight, I would have chosen different options as my first line of defense. I've learned that there are places where people go with cancer that is deemed terminal and, after weeks of alternative care and treatment, return home cancer-free. This is worth your time and quality of life, but you must reclaim your power and do your research.

I have followed much of what is in this handbook to assist me in my recovery, and I am confident to say that it has saved my life and given me many more quality years. I wish you peace, joy, and laughter today and always… Hugs to your heart, Ron Baron.